DOUG DE GROOD

THE RIGHT SIDE OF THE FAIRWAY

ISBN 13: 979-860175564-1

Printed in the United States of America
24   23   22   21   20   5   4   3   2   1

Cover design by Heidi Konkel
Interior design by James Monroe Design, LLC.

For Mom, the most positive form of energy I'll ever know
and
Michaelanne, my Maine squeeze for 25 years
and the best cancer drug money can't buy.

Praise for *THE RIGHT SIDE OF THE FAIRWAY*

"This is one of the most poignant, insightful, witty and frank perspectives on dealing with cancer I have come across. This should be required reading not only for people faced with this life-threatening condition and their families, but also doctors, nurses and all others involved in supporting these courageous individuals (even the non-golfers)."

—Badrinath Konety, MD

"Doug deGrood writes as a mature believer—one who has learned that our faith doesn't promise that we'll never suffer but rather that suffering and challenges in life can ultimately bring us closer to God. In the end, the path to glory is the path of descent, knowing that God is with us every step of the way. And for that, the only appropriate response is gratitude."

—Fr. Michael Reding, Pastor, St. Thomas the Apostle

CONTENTS

CONTENTS

INTRODUCTION

In the spring of 2015, not long after my 50th birthday and in the prime of my life, I was diagnosed with urothelial carcinoma, or bladder cancer. When I shared the unwelcome news with family and friends in an email, I referred to my diagnosis as a "double bogey." I used that particular metaphor because not only am I a certifiable golfoholic, but the best round of golf I ever played started, ironically enough, with a double bogey. So why couldn't I expect the same result this time around with cancer? Why couldn't my diagnosis, while as unwelcome as the shanks, lead to something great?

The following pages offer my thoughts and perspective on life with cancer through the lens of golf. For those hoping to find some silver bullet for conquering the disease, you will be sadly disappointed. I'm not sure one exists. But you will find validation of some powerful, universal truths, many of which you might already be aware but not fully appreciative.

Golf, like life, is a funny game. You never know how the ball's going to bounce. Good shots are sometimes penalized, and bad shots are miraculously rewarded. In the end, what matters is your attitude and how you deal with the cards you're dealt. If you expect the worst, fearing the hazards lining the fairways, more times than not, that's where you'll end up. But if you focus on the short grass and expect the best, you just might find yourself sitting pretty with a nice little flip wedge into a big, welcoming green.

So what's it going to be? That, my friends, is entirely up to you. Let's tee it up, shall we?

PART 1

THE FRONT NINE

1

THAT'S THE WAY THE OL' BALL BOUNCES

You're standing on the tee of a par-3 hole with water in front. You confidently step up, stick your peg in the ground, place your ball so the logo is pointing just so. You methodically go through your pre-shot routine, envision the perfect shot, and with total commitment, you pull the trigger and make rock-solid contact.

As you stand there posing, the ball takes off on a promising trajectory. It's literally tracing the shot pattern you drew up in your mind a moment ago. You're already thinking about buying everyone in the clubhouse drinks to celebrate your ace. That is, until a sudden gust of wind comes up. Your ball, which had been on autopilot, now starts to balloon. It rises higher and higher and now seems to be moving backward. As it starts its descent, you're now out of your picture-perfect pose and into the fetal position, praying your ball clears the water. But your prayer goes unanswered as your ball, which five seconds ago was destined for the cup, lands a millimeter short of clearing the last rock at the edge of the pond, ricochets high into the air, and splashes down in a watery grave. Congratulations. You're now hitting three.

Next, your playing partner steps up. He almost trips as he sticks his tee in the ground. He takes a couple grotesque practice swings, then hits a cold hard hosel rocket. Ducks scatter as his ball skims across the pond, skipping five times before colliding with the same rock your ball hit moments ago. But instead of deflecting backward, it pops high into the air and lands as softly as a butterfly with sore feet five feet from the pin.

Could someone please explain the justice in this?

In the spring of 2015, I had just turned 50 and was feeling on top of the world. My business partner and I had just sold our successful ad agency. Unlike most men my age, my stomach was still flat thanks to a daily regimen of sit-ups and push-ups. I had an ideal BMI of 22. My blood pressure and cholesterol were both excellent. I didn't smoke. The only time I'd been hospitalized was the day I was born. I was the very picture of health. Or so I thought.

That May, I happened to be in Atlanta attending my niece's wedding. After the reception, I went to use the bathroom in my hotel room and peed what can only be described as a reddish-brown mélange of... well, I'll spare you the details. After returning home to Minneapolis the next day, I called my friend Dr. Dan Dunn and explained my symptoms. We scheduled a CT scan, which unfortunately revealed polyps. Dan tried to calm my fears, telling me that most bladder tumors are either benign or highly treatable. But he also prepared me for the worst. I then had a cystoscopy, which is like a colonoscopy, except the tiny camera enters "the front door." I was watching the video screen with the urologist as he went spelunking in my bladder. And that's when we saw them: two grotesque critters attached to the wall of my bladder. We didn't know much about them at this stage. Were they harmless growths, or were they malignant monsters bent on widespread destruction? All I knew for certain was I wanted them out.

Surgery was scheduled for the following month. My family had our annual summer trip to Maine scheduled the next week, and my doctor saw no reason to cancel it. I took that as a good sign. If he had been worried, he'd have wanted to operate immediately, right? What's more, I had done enough research to know that bladder cancer doesn't carry with it the death sentence of some other cancers.

A week later, I underwent endoscopic surgery to remove what we thought would be two small tumors. It turned out there were four, and one of them was highly aggressive—carcinoma in situ. It grows like moss, so its borders are hard to define and, as a result, remove.

The surgeon got good margins, which showed no muscle invasion. Phew! We caught it early—stage I. My treatment plan called for six weeks of BCG therapy, which stands for Bacillus Calmette-Guerin. It's a type of topical immunotherapy that involves placing a weakened form of the tuberculosis virus in your bladder through a catheter. You leave it in for two hours, then pee it out. It's intended to stimulate your immune system to go after the bad guys, and it's up to seventy percent effective. How can you not like those odds? Answer: when you're in the thirty percent who don't respond.

My tumors came back, so we did more surgery, followed by six more weeks of BCG therapy. Biopsy surgery would later confirm if indeed the second time was the charm. And to the naked eye, things had improved. Unfortunately, the pathology report told a different story. Not only was cancer still present, but it had now invaded the muscle tissue—stage II. Time to remove the bladder.

Talk about a stretch of bad holes. And the worst part was I felt like I had done everything right. I prayed with the fervor of Job. I had made significant changes to my diet, including mostly giving up alcohol (no easy feat for this scotch whisky lover). I did self-guided meditation and worked really hard at reducing stress. I even went to see a Reiki healer!

Sitting in the waiting room of the cancer clinic added to my frustration. I would frequently witness morbidly obese people sneaking outside to have a smoke. Based on conventional health wisdom, I understood why these people might be sick. I'm not suggesting they deserved it. But why was I sick? The whole experience was hard on my ego, not to mention my faith.

It was then I came to accept the fact that those are the breaks in life. You can execute a great golf shot only to have it foiled by a gust of wind or a funny bounce. It doesn't mean you deserved it any more than it means you deserved the good break you received on the previous hole when you hit a poor tee shot, a poor second shot, and then holed a long bunker shot for birdie.

This is arguably the toughest lesson of cancer: coming to terms with the sometimes-indiscriminate nature of it. Yes, there are lots of smokers who get cancer. But there are plenty of nonsmokers who get it as well. Much has been written about why bad things happen to good people. The fact is, lightning can strike one person just as easily as the next. There's simply no room for retributive justice in nature. The natural, human inclination when dealt a bum hand—even among people of faith—is to conclude God must be punishing us for some prior sin. But I don't believe God punishes people. Nor does he reward them. He simply loves us, and that love—if we accept it—gives us the strength to shoulder life's inevitable burdens.

The popular refrain at the cancer pity party is "Why me?" I suggest turning that question around and asking instead, "Why not me?" As in, why shouldn't you be the one who defies the odds and overcomes cancer? After all, somebody has to. Give me one good reason why it shouldn't be you.

2

WHEN IN DOUBT, LOOSEN YOUR GRIP PRESSURE

Whenever I'm playing golf with someone whose game is going sideways, I always suggest they try easing up on their grip pressure. This usually results in them hurling a few choice expletives at me. But after they calm down, they usually try it, and voilà, their swing is magically restored.

Easing up on your grip pressure is the duct tape of golf remedies: it fixes anything. By letting go a little, we actually regain the control we lost when we were trying to squeeze the golf club into submission. Rhythm and flow—essential elements of a good golf swing—are magically restored.

The same can be true in life. Before I was diagnosed with cancer, I was definitely guilty of gripping too tight. Most of my friends would never suspect it, but I was a closet worrywart. My public persona was laid-back, happy-go-lucky. But underneath, I had a lot of pent-up anxiety. The ad agency I worked at, of which I was a founding partner, had a mantra that we actually trademarked: Always Thinking®. Looking back, it's clear I took these words a little too much to heart. I was constantly waking up in the middle of the night, my mind racing with any number of work-related thoughts. When I couldn't get back to sleep, I'd go downstairs to my study, get on my computer, and fire off emails. People who received these nocturnal missives would frequently notice the time at which they were sent and make jokes about my unusual office hours. It got so bad I had to send a memo to our entire company letting them know I wasn't a vampire, and just because I was working at three in the morning didn't mean I expected them to keep the same hours.

After I was diagnosed with cancer, my grip didn't exactly ease up. I read all the popular books about coping with cancer, did countless hours of online research, joined online chat groups. I was totally preoccupied with my illness. And that's not always a good thing. It's like having too many swing thoughts in golf. You become too mechanical and stop doing what comes naturally.

And here's the other thing: I was relying too much on Doug to dig myself out of the hole I was in. I had taken my eye off the ball. I lost sight of my faith and the fact that I'm not alone, that there is a higher power, and for me, that power is God. If I just let go a little—acknowledge my vulnerability—I could tap into God's saving grace and start healing. Throughout this book, I'll touch on some of the ways I've learned to let go and tap into that power.

Meditation—An Enema for Your Brain

I discovered meditation to be incredibly effective at clearing out noisy thoughts. Of course, when many people hear the word meditation, they think patchouli oil and sitar music. Or they're confused as to what exactly it is. I think of it essentially as being more mindful of your breathing. In yogi culture, it's believed we're all given a limited number of breaths, so naturally, you want to make the most of them. YouTube offers a treasure trove of self-guided meditation videos. I highly recommend the ones narrated by Australians. There's something about the Aussie accent that's very soothing, especially when spoken slowly in hushed tones. There are also meditation apps like Headspace. The key is to make it part of your daily routine. Think of it like showering, but for your soul. It helps to set an alarm or put it on your Outlook calendar. Ten minutes is all it takes, which is far less time-consuming than going to the gym and, I would argue, just as beneficial. Meditation reduces stress, which causes inflammation. It improves sleep. And it can even make you a kinder person. What's more, you can do it anywhere, anytime. So take a breather. And breathe.

Don't Worry, Be Healthy

I almost feel ashamed when I think back to some of the things I used to consider important. Living with a life-threatening disease has a way of doing that. Today, trivial concerns—tomorrow's big meeting, Roth versus traditional IRAs— go to bed when I do. I've learned the hard way they're not worth losing sleep. Worse, I believe worry can cause real harm, not only mentally and emotionally, but physically, too.

I have no empirical data to support this, but I believe one of the leading causes of cancer isn't smoking or poor diet. It's stress. I think there's more to the expression "What's eating you?" than we know. I believe that anxiety can literally eat away at our insides until the next thing you know, you're in a hotel room in Atlanta for your niece's wedding and... well, you already know that story.

Letting Go of Our Stuff

Inscribed on U.S. currency in all caps are the words IN GOD WE TRUST. I've always found this ironic: our money reminds us not to place too much value on our money. And yet from time to time, most of us are guilty of gripping too tightly to material things.

I don't think I'd ever be accused of being a "showy" person. I live in a modest home, drive a modest car. But there are times when I allow my possessions to possess me, falsely believing they'll bring me security, rather than trusting in God's grace. Material wealth and its promise of happiness is a powerful illusion. And so we keep accumulating stuff. But it never makes us any happier. Inevitably, our stuff lets us down. You're probably familiar with the expression, "The most important things in life aren't things." As much as I like to poke fun at millennials, they seem to get this concept more so than my generation.

Of course, it isn't just stuff that can possess us. Things like social media, FOMO (fear of missing out), TV binge watching, alcohol, sweets, or any number of vices can quickly take control of our lives. The good news is that as easy as it is to become captive to these things, freeing ourselves is equally simple (albeit difficult): just lighten your grip pressure. Let go. Stop obsessing. Or, as my Apple Watch is constantly reminding me, "Breathe."

The band .38 Special probably said it best: "Just hold on loosely, but don't let go. If you cling too tightly, you're gonna lose control."

3

IT'S A STREAKY GAME

Is there any game more fickle than golf? At times, it seems so easy, like you've got it all figured out. You'll go on a hot streak and rattle off half a dozen great rounds in a row and watch your handicap plummet. And then, without warning and for no apparent reason, things change for the worse. You lose that lovin' feelin' and the game is a struggle.

Streaks are a funny thing. They're so... streaky. But one thing we know for certain: All streaks come to an end eventually, no matter how hot or cold. They're like weather patterns.

When I was originally diagnosed with bladder cancer, I had no idea what I was in for. Would it be a short-term bump in the road? Or would it be time to start planning my funeral? At the time, my urologist was optimistic. But the series of events that ensued were far from rosy.

The following is a recap of the worst losing streak of my life:

July 2015

It started with my original biopsy surgery, which revealed multiple tumors, including carcinoma in situ, a highly aggressive cancer. If that weren't bad enough, the internal bleeding from my biopsy surgery got so bad I had to be rushed to the emergency room and hospitalized.

Once I recovered, I started on BCG therapy, which I described earlier. My treatments were every week for six weeks. The side effects were unpleasant but manageable. In addition to a burning sensation, it also caused bladder tissue to slough off and get discharged in my urine, which I elegantly described to friends as "peeing ground beef." Sorry, I know, too much information, or as my kids say, TMI.

After my six-week cycle, I had a second biopsy surgery. Unfortunately, the tumors had grown back, so we scheduled six more weeks of BCG therapy, followed by a third biopsy surgery and more bad news. Not only was the disease still present, but it had progressed into the muscle lining, which is considered stage II cancer. I thought, no big deal, we'll just remove my bladder, and that'll be that! I wasn't exactly happy about losing my bladder. I had grown rather attached to it over the years. But compared to the alternative, it seemed like a small price to pay.

March 2016

Before surgery, I had to undergo chemotherapy to try to shrink the cancer. Because of my relatively young age and good health, my oncologist pulled no punches— he prescribed MVAC, which stands for Methotrexate, Vinblastine, Adriamycin, and Cisplatin. This is about as heavy-duty as chemo gets. My infusions lasted eight hours, and because of the high level of toxicity, they needed to be spaced every other week. I experienced the usual side effects: nausea, fatigue, occasional vomiting. I lost my hair, which really wasn't such a bad experience. I marveled at my ability to shower in under two minutes. Hair, it turns out, is a nuisance. Although it does do quite a good job of keeping your head warm in the winter. Worse was when I lost my taste for scotch. And in the cruelest of ironies, what do you suppose everyone gave me as a "get well" gift? That's right, enough single malt scotch to flood a small wading pool.

June 2016

The surgery I opted for—radical cystectomy with neobladder reconstruction—involves the removal of your bladder and the construction of a new one using a two-foot chunk of your small intestine. They remove your prostate at the same time since the two organs work in tandem. So at least I won't have to worry about prostate cancer! This particular surgery is considered one of the toughest because it impacts two major systems of your anatomy—urinary and gastrointestinal. I'm not ashamed to admit it totally kicked my butt. I lost twenty pounds and was noticeably weak for months. I took a two-month medical leave from work and used every minute.

I should point out that life with a neobladder is different. Because it lacks the nerve endings of your factory bladder, you don't experience the sensation of "needing to go," which makes it necessary to set a timer to remind yourself to empty your bladder every three to four hours, day and night.

A few weeks after surgery, I had a follow-up appointment where I received some news that took my breath away. While the autopsy of my bladder showed the lymph nodes were cancer-free, they did find the disease in a couple lymph nodes in my belly. In other words, the genie was out of the bottle. I had stage IV metastatic bladder cancer. This is somewhat rare for the cancer to skip from one organ to another part of the body. But what can I say, I'm unique.

Because my body was technically cancer-free at that point in time, they couldn't prescribe any additional treatment. All we could do was wait. Or, if I was willing, I could take part in a yearlong drug trial they were conducting at the University of Minnesota for a relatively new immunotherapy drug, known commercially as Opdivo. There was a catch, though. It was a double-blind study, so there was a fifty-fifty chance I'd get the drug or the placebo, and we wouldn't know for twelve months. My doctors and nurses wouldn't even know. I figured, what could it hurt? At best, I'd get the drug and it might prevent my cancer from coming back. At worst, I'd be helping advance medical science, which would bring good karma. And so I became a guinea pig.

September 2016

Because I was going to get stuck with a needle every other week for the next fifty-two weeks, my trial manager, Kate, suggested I get an IV port. It's a device about the size of a Starburst candy that's surgically implanted in your chest. It allows nurses to access your veins with a tiny needle instead of fishing around in your arm or hand with a big needle. As much as I disliked the idea of going under the knife, the prospect of looking like a heroin addict swayed me to get the port.

And so every other week, I'd visit Kate and my new family at the University of Minnesota Southdale Cancer Clinic. Because you end up spending so much time with these people, they become family. My wife, Michaelanne, referred to Kate as my cancer wife. She was a godsend. We'd talk and laugh. She'd score me free parking in the hospital ramp, free coupons for Ensure. If I ever needed to contact my urologist or oncologist, she'd have them on the line in minutes. It was like having my own personal medical concierge.

August 2017

During the trial, I continued to have CT scans every twelve weeks. I had nearly completed my twelfth and final month of treatment when a scan revealed that my cancer had spread. They immediately unblinded me from the study, and to my surprise (and relief), I had been receiving the placebo.

Before going any further, I decided to get a second opinion at the Mayo Clinic, which is just an hour and a half south of Minneapolis. The doctors there confirmed the recommendations of my doctors at the University of Minnesota that I should immediately start immunotherapy treatment with the drug Keytruda.

But Wait, There's More...

I forgot to point out that not long after my neo-bladder surgery, I started contracting urinary tract infections (UTIs) on a fairly frequent basis. This is somewhat common in people with neobladders. I'd get really bad chills and night sweats. Antibiotics would usually wipe it out in a few days, but in the meantime, I would have to huddle under a thick wool blanket wearing multiple layers of clothing.

At first, the UTIs would occur every four to five weeks. Then they started happening more frequently: every three weeks, then every two weeks. This made life, and especially traveling, difficult, since I never knew when an infection might come on. This went on for a year, at which point I started working with an infectious disease doctor who prescribed a daily regimen of methenamine. It's not technically an antibiotic, but it works like one. It converts to formaldehyde in your bladder, which kills bacteria.

This helped some, but UTIs still persisted. Worse, I started noticing small particles of food in my urine, things like lettuce, spinach, even tomato seeds. So I did what all genius health advocates do: I went on the internet and self-diagnosed—with a fair degree of certainty, I might add—that I had a fistula between my neobladder and my lower bowel. A fistula is an abnormal connection between two body parts. When I suggested this to my urologist, Dr. Konety—a nationally renowned urologic surgeon and the director of the Institute for Prostate and Urologic Cancers at the University of Minnesota—he gave me the look any doctor gives a patient who's been spending too much time on WebMD. But he ordered an X-ray of my bladder, and sure enough, I was right. Any giddiness I might have experienced from being vindicated was quickly snuffed out by the fact that I had a fistula!

How it happened is anyone's guess, but it was likely caused by a surgery staple. I could live with the abnormality, but my colorectal surgeon, Dr. Madoff, recommended that if I was planning on living to a ripe old age, I should have it fixed, which would require major surgery. Of course, the answer to that question hinged on how I would respond to the immunotherapy treatments.

In case you're keeping score, here's where we're at:

- Transurethral resection of bladder tumors—revealed stage I disease

- Two six-week cycles of BCG therapy—failed

- Chemo—failed

- Radical cystectomy—Performed too late to prevent cancer from becoming metastatic

- 12-month drug study—Received the placebo

- Developed a rare fistula which caused chronic UTIs.

Talk about a cold streak. I had grown so accustomed to bad news I was numb to it. Which is what made the good news that finally came all the more surprising. After just one 12-week cycle of immunotherapy, I had a strong positive response. My PET scan revealed significant reduction in the size of the diseased lymph nodes. After the next cycle, the results were even better. This continued for three more cycles when my oncologist, Dr. Gupta, uttered the words every cancer patient longs to hear, "You've had a complete response." The streak had ended.

To put this in context, the type of immunotherapy treatment I received has a response rate of about 29 percent. Which means only one in three experience some kind of benefit. And of those 29 percent, less than half will have a "complete response," meaning there is no visible sign of disease in the body.

As of December 2019, I've been cancer-free for nearly two years. I stopped treatments in September 2018, one year after I started them. I felt bullish enough about the future that I went ahead and had surgery to repair my fistula, which was no picnic. It required a ten-inch incision in my lower abdomen, which took six weeks to heal. I'll continue to get scanned every twelve weeks for the foreseeable future. If I stay cancer-free for five years, I'll be considered "cured."

I guess you could say I'm currently on a hot streak.

4

IT'S A GAME OF OPPOSITES

I believe one of the biggest reasons people find golf so difficult is because it's so counterintuitive. You make the ball fade to the *right* by swinging inside to the *left* (if you're right-handed). You generate clubhead speed by making the clubhead lag behind in your backswing. You propel the ball *up* into the air by striking it *down* into the ground.

I've always found this last paradox especially profound. How often do we rise only after falling? Remember learning to ride a bike? Or maybe you failed at one job for which you were ill-suited, only to have that lead you to another career in which you could flourish. Of course, the ultimate example is the story of Jesus, who achieved ultimate glory by dying on a cross. I know we're getting deep into the fescue here, but it's a universal truth: only by dying a little do we ultimately live.

I often think of life as being like a round of golf, with front and back nines. The front nine is all about rising. You go to school, get a job, work hard, play by the rules and reap the rewards for having done all the right things. The back nine is all about falling. Parents who were once there to tend to our needs now need someone to tend to them. Small kids with small problems are now big kids with big problems. Addiction, illness, any number of crises arise, beating us down into the ground. And yet it's these dark moments that are actually illuminating the path to a better understanding of the meaning of life and the concept of hope and God's mercy.

Father Richard Rohr, a Franciscan friar from Albuquerque, New Mexico, writes brilliantly about this subject in his book *Falling Upward*. I highly recommend it to anyone currently on the back nine of life.

Humble Piety

One of my favorite passages from Luke's Gospel is "He who exalts himself shall be humbled, and he who humbles himself shall be exalted." How many times have we seen this play out in real life? Our current president and many of his former campaign staff come to mind.

One by one, they seem to be trading in their pinstripes for orange jumpsuits. Compare that to the news stories about the secret millionaire next door. The one who eschewed the spotlight only to leave his or her entire fortune to some worthy cause. Who's the rock star now?

The Money Paradox

When my kids ask me for career advice, I always tell them the same thing: never take a job for the money. Do what you love, and you'll love what you do. The money part will sort itself out. "Huh? You mean I'll make more money if I set aside money as the objective?" In a word, yes. Making money is not the purpose of a person or a business, truly successful ones anyway. Their purpose needs to be higher. And if that purpose is achieved, the money inevitably follows. In fact, the moment you choose money as your goal is the moment you take your eyes off the ball of what made you happy and successful in the first place, which inevitably leads to a decline in performance and, ironically enough, money.

The Virtues of Benign Neglect

One of my greatest fears as a parent today is that we're robbing our kids of their initiative. From helicopter parenting to indulging their every material desire, many of us are smoothing out far too many bumps in the road before our young people. It's these very bumps that build character and produce successful adults. Any psychologist will tell you young people need to be given permission to fail. If they're not failing, they're neither pushing the boundaries nor learning how to deal with disappointment. The funny thing is, pretty much everyone I know grew up in what I would characterize as a state of benign neglect. We were latchkey children. Our parents didn't attend every hockey game. They didn't pay for spring break trips. But as parents of our own kids, some of us have swung hard in the opposite direction. Many of us feel compelled to lavish them with stuff, protect them from sharp objects whenever possible. But by doing so, our kids can become dull.

When I was a kid, I really wanted a Crosman pellet gun. I asked my mom if she would buy it for me. She told me no, but suggested I might earn the money by going door-to-door selling tomatoes from our vegetable garden. I didn't like her idea very much, but I really wanted that pellet gun. So I loaded up our little red wagon with big red tomatoes and somehow mustered the courage to become the youngest greengrocer in the history of Bloomington, Minnesota. In a way, I'm still selling tomatoes today.

Care Less. Enjoy More.

In golf, how many times have you scored better by not caring about your score? I remember one round in particular several years ago. I showed up just as my group was teeing off on the first hole. Without any warm-up or even a single practice swing, I stepped up and hit my drive right down the middle. A few hours later, as I was lining up a putt on the 18th hole, one of my buddies said to me, "You know, if you make this, you'll shoot 74." I couldn't believe it. I knew I had been hitting the ball well, but I hadn't been keeping score. I was just enjoying myself, not thinking. And yes, there might have been a few beers involved. Needless to say, I didn't make the putt, but I did two-putt for par and a 75. Not too shabby for a high single-digit handicap.

5

RAIN MAKES THE GRASS GROW

There's nothing more disappointing to a golfer than looking forward excitedly to a round of golf only to have the weather rain on your parade. And yet without that rain, there'd be no golf course and, therefore, no golf. (I realize this logic doesn't apply in the Arizona desert, where irrigation practices are literally changing weather patterns.) The point being seemingly negative events can bring about positive outcomes.

There is perhaps no finer redemption story in the history of golf than that of Eldrick "Tiger" Woods. Tiger first achieved stardom as a club-toting toddler on "The Mike Douglas Show" in 1978. I don't need to tell you what happened next. Even people who think a wedge is a hunk of iceberg lettuce drizzled with balsamic are familiar with the Tiger Woods story. While he's still three majors short of Jack Nicklaus's record of eighteen majors, an argument can be made that Tiger is the greatest of all time. He won three U.S. Amateurs in a row, which is two more than Jack. He has more PGA Tour wins than Jack. And, I would argue, the pool of elite competitors is deeper today than it was in Jack's era.

Not too many years ago, it was a foregone conclusion in most experts' minds—Mr. Nicklaus's included—that Tiger would eclipse Jack's record for major wins. But then the rains started to fall. Not long after he somehow managed to win the 2008 U.S. Open on one leg, his dark secret about a life of infidelity was revealed in the tabloids, costing him his marriage and his reputation. That was followed by chronic back issues which hampered his ability to swing a golf club, eroding his legendary confidence and mythical aura. In May of 2017, he was arrested on suspicion of driving under the influence of painkillers. He later sought treatment for opioid addiction. By July 2017, he had fallen out of the top 1,000 in the Official World Golf Rankings. Tiger's career seemed all but over.

Full disclosure: I've never been a member of the Tiger fan club. Of course, I have the utmost respect for his game and everything he's accomplished. But golf fandom is binary: you're either a Tiger guy or a Phil Mickelson guy, and I like Lefty. That said, I sympathize with what Tiger's been through the past decade. The personal demons he's battled under intense public scrutiny and ridicule you wouldn't wish on anyone. And yet all these setbacks appear to have had a positive effect on him. He smiles more. He seems more comfortable in his skin, more affable, less aloof. He seems to have developed a sense of humility. Even his trademark fist pump is kinder-looking.

In September 2018, Tiger captured the Tour Championship, putting himself back in the winner's circle for the first time in five years. And then, in April 2019, Tiger completed his comeback, winning his fifth Masters with a performance as brilliant as Augusta National's famous azaleas. The roar is definitely back. And to think just one year earlier, there was serious doubt whether he'd ever play competitive golf again. For the first time in my life, I'm a Tiger Woods fan.

The Gift of Cancer

Those who know me will tell you I'm hardly shy about sharing my thoughts and opinions. Throughout my career in advertising, I was known as something of a provocateur. My MO was shoot first, ask questions later; I thought I had all the answers. At times, that confidence might have even bordered on arrogance.

The success that followed only served to reinforce that my shit must not stink. I was named a Creative All-Star by ADWEEK magazine when I was in my mid-twenties. The agency I co-founded was twice named the most creative small agency in America by the American Association of Ad Agencies. My business partner and I sold our company in 2015, providing a level of financial security. I thought I had it all. But then my own rains came, in the form of cancer.

I remember my friend Char, a fellow cancer survivor, coming to visit me after my diagnosis, telling me that cancer brings all sorts of changes, some of which are actually quite positive. While I couldn't fully appreciate what she meant at the time, I quickly came to understand. I think it's fair to say that cancer has changed me for the better. I've become less sharp with my tongue, slower to anger. I'm a better listener, more understanding of people with different points of view. I feel much more at peace. I'm less hurried, taking more time to stop and appreciate the world around me. I'm more appreciative of people in my life. And to think all it took was a life-threatening illness.

Life After Cancer

I've always been a work-before-play kind of person. Because of my practical nature, I found it hard to splurge on exotic trips or indulgences. I kept telling myself I would do that stuff once I retired. But cancer is incredibly effective at reminding you of how important it is to live in the now, that there might not be a tomorrow. Today, I'm much more inclined to spontaneously go out to that cool new restaurant, see a show, or say yes to a guys' golf trip. Would I have preferred not to get cancer? Yes. But am I enjoying life more now than before cancer? Yes.

6

THE ONLY THING WORSE THAN BAD GOLF IS NO GOLF

In April 2016, I had plans to attend my annual guys' golf weekend, affectionately known as the Curly Rough Invitational. That year marked our 21st anniversary, and we were headed to Pinehurst, North Carolina. If you've been there, you know how magical, almost mystical, a place it is. Located in Sandhills country in the middle of the state (and the middle of nowhere really), it is a true destination. Nearly everyone is there to gouge divots from some of the most hallowed ground in golf-dom—Donald Ross's famed Pinehurst #2. I was right in the middle of my chemotherapy treatments, but I hadn't missed a single Curly Rough in 21 years, and I wasn't going to start now.

I figured at worst, I might have to skip a few holes if fatigue became an issue. But it didn't, thanks in part to the steroids my oncologist prescribed. I did have a few bouts of nausea. But the excitement and enjoyment of playing golf provided an effective tonic. In fact, that weekend I drove the ball straighter and longer than I have in my entire life. Maybe it was the steroids. (Good thing no one asked me to pee in a cup!) Unfortunately, I had the exact opposite luck with my short game. My nerves were super shaky. Hole after hole, I'd have a wedge or short iron in, and I couldn't hit the broad side of a barn. After missing the green, I'd lay the sod over a couple chip shots and yip a few putts before one of my buddies would mercifully say, "That's good."

My scores were humiliating, and I pretty much shot myself out of contention of winning the coveted Curly Rough gold blazer on day one. But I didn't care. Despite my competitive nature, I adjusted my expectations, and score didn't matter. I found plenty of satisfaction walking the golf courses and hitting the occasional good shot. Not to mention I was playing golf with my friends in the warm sunshine, not stuck back in the wintry cold of Minnesota.

Four weeks later, having finished my chemo treatments, I managed to join another group of golfing buddies on a trip to Barton Creek in Austin, Texas. My scores were equally miserable, but the way I looked at it, it was Doug 2, cancer 0.

A Simple Choice

When you have a terminal illness like cancer, or any major setback for that matter, it's easy to become consumed by it, to let it dominate your thoughts and prevent you from living. You get sucked into a black hole of darkness and fear. And the more you wallow in the darkness, the deeper you descend into the abyss.

At one particularly low point during my illness, I made a conscious decision to stop buying new clothes. I concluded if there's a chance I'm going to die sooner rather than later, why fritter away money on clothes I won't be able to wear? This is partly the result of my frugal Dutch DNA. But still, can you get any more defeatist?! It was at this point I was reminded of a line from my favorite movie, *The Shawshank Redemption*: "Get busy living or get busy dying."

In the end, whether you have a terminal illness or not, isn't that what it all comes down to? After all, only God knows how long we're going to live, and he's not telling. Any one of us could get hit by a bus tomorrow. There's a difference between living and merely breathing. Here are some of the ways I choose to live.

- Playing my trumpet
- Listening to music (classical, jazz, and alternative rock)
- Reading

- Watching documentary films
- Playing golf or tennis
- Going for long walks in the woods
- Pulling weeds in the garden
- Watching birds and pollinators in my backyard
- Riding my bike to a nearby lake and going fishing
- Puttering around on my backyard putting green
- Cutting the grass
- Spending time with other humans
- Writing this book

When I'm engaged in these activities, the last thing I'm thinking about is my mortality. After all, I'm up to my eyeballs in life. It's like a Jedi mind trick. Okay, maybe not that cool, but equally effective. The point is, living is a conscious decision. And that decision is easier to make when you have something to live for.

7

THE GRASS IS RARELY GREENER ON THE OTHER SIDE

The golf industry loves to prey on human weakness. Can you blame it? We're all a bunch of head cases. The answer to a better swing, more distance, and lower scores is always just an equipment change away. An insatiable appetite for the latest and greatest needs to be fed, and we have no qualms indulging it. After all, it's not the carpenter; it's the tools! We buy into this fallacy knowing full well that long term, our scores aren't going to improve much. It does, however, make for good small talk on the golf course.

"Hey, I see you got the new MegaTron driver. How do you like it?"

"Oh, I love it. Best driver I've ever had. I'm hitting the ball farther, straighter, and I've even started to regrow my hair!"

I've always resisted the temptation to change equipment, mostly because it requires opening my wallet, which I don't like to do. But also because my mother didn't raise a fool! Prior to my current set of TaylorMade irons, now nine years old, I had a set of Ping Eye 2 irons that I purchased in 1988 and played for twenty-two years. At one point, I even sent them back to the Ping factory to have them sandblasted and refinished.

I play golf with a guy who still putts with a brass Bullseye putter, and he's one of the better putters I know. While the rest of the world continually experiments with various lengths and styles of putters, different grips, postures, etc., he reduces the number of variables. One putter. One stroke. There are never any surprises. He might be hotter some days than others, but overall, his putting is a model of consistency. And so are his scores.

Most people, however, are not wired this way. We believe the grass is always greener. I see it frequently in men and women my age who decide suddenly, after twenty-plus years of marriage and raising a bunch of great kids, they'd be happier if they traded in their current life for a new one, complete with a new partner, new home, new car, new wardrobe, new everything. Once the "new car smell" wears off, I wonder, how many of them are actually happier?

I'm not being judgmental or suggesting that people should stay in toxic or abusive relationships. I'm actually quite sympathetic. We're only human, and by nature, we're rarely satisfied. No matter how much money we have, how big our houses, how fancy our vacations, it's never enough. That is, until we embrace the concept of gratitude. Maybe you've seen one of those little wooden plaques in somebody's kitchen: "Gratitude turns what we have into enough." I know I shouldn't be looking to HomeGoods for philosophy lessons, but it's true.

It starts when we're little kids. "She got more ice cream than me!" From that point on, we keep comparing our stuff to other people's stuff, which leads to envy and even animosity. Social media and the constant flaunting of "winning" exacerbates the problem. No wonder teen depression and suicide rates are at an all-time high.

A Thankful Heart Is a Happy Heart

On my drive to work in the morning, I'm in the habit of saying out loud, in the privacy of my car so people don't think I'm a nut, "Thanks be to God." That's it. Four simple words that somehow manage to make a complex world simple and put a smile on my face. By reciting these four simple words, I'm reminded of the countless things I have to be thankful for, and that everything I have comes from God. They're usually small things with little or no intrinsic value, like the sunrise, or the person who let me merge in front of them on the highway entrance ramp, or heated car seats in January in Minnesota.

By taking great pleasure in little things and being in the habit of thanking God for them, I've discovered it takes less and less to make me truly happy. A glass of single malt, a comfortable chair, a little Rachmaninoff playing on the stereo, and I'm in heaven. Don't get me wrong, I'm not saying I wouldn't derive immense enjoyment from, say, belonging to Pine Valley or Cypress Point. But I don't need it to be fulfilled either.

Less Is More, More or Less

My wife's grandmother, Sis Kelm, was an amazing woman. Technically, she was my wife's step-grandmother, but if she were alive, she'd scold me for saying that. She had an amazing capacity to love. She had been married three times. Her first husband had three children by a previous marriage. She gave birth to two children of her own. After two more marriages, late in life, she acquired several more stepchildren and step-grandchildren. But in her mind, they were all either out of her womb or out of her heart, and she truly did not make any distinction between the two.

She was a more willowy version of Barbara Bush, with perfectly coiffed white hair and an irresistible Virginia accent. She had this go-to phrase whenever a waiter or waitress at a restaurant asked if we wanted anything else: "Elegant sufficiency. Any more would be an abundance." I love that expression, so much so that I stole it and use it on a regular basis. Not only does it keep this great woman alive in my heart, but it's a powerful reminder to me and those around me that enough really is enough.

8

GOLF CAN BE HELL.
BUT IT'S A DRY HEAT.

We've all heard the expression: a bad round of golf is better than a good day at the office. Most golfers would agree. Although I've had a few rounds that challenge this axiom. One in particular came at TPC Scottsdale. It was so bad I nearly quit golf and took up tennis. (No offense to my tennis-playing friends.) Early in the round, I came down with a case of the shanks. On one hole, I needed five shots to get out of a greenside bunker. I was playing in a stroke-play tournament and didn't have the option of simply picking up my ball and taking my max score. I made a ten on the hole en route to shooting a hundred-something.

The reality is, we all have bad days, and some are worse than others. One day I'll never forget: February

29, 2016. The fact that it was Leap Day already made it memorable. I renamed it "Leap of Faith Day" for reasons that will soon become obvious. On this auspicious day, I had my social security number stolen, the result of a data breach at our company; I learned my son, who'd been battling a mysterious autoimmune disease for the past five years, might now have cancer (which later turned out to be a false alarm); and I was given the bad news by my doctor that my cancer had progressed to stage II, and as a result, I would need to have my bladder and prostate removed.

They say bad things come in threes, and this day certainly proved it. I only wish my unholy trinity could have been comprised of lesser tragedies, like a speeding ticket or a hangnail. And yet as bad as things were, I had to laugh. I mean, seriously, could my life get any worse? The answer, painfully, is yes.

No matter how bad things are, they can always be worse. When I remind myself of that, it never fails to make me feel better. A nice, deep sigh usually helps too. There's a great song in the Broadway hit *Seussical the Musical* that expands on this theme:

> When the news is all bad
> When you're sour and blue
> When you start to get mad
> You should do what I do
> Tell yourself how lucky you are…

When your life's going wrong
When the fates are unkind
When you're limping along
And get kicked from behind
Tell yourself how lucky you are...

Why decry a cloudy sky?
An empty purse?
A crazy universe?
My philosophy is simply
Things could be worse!

So be happy you're here
Think of life as a thrill
And if worse comes to worse
As we all know it will
Thank your lucky star
You've gotten this far...
Tell yourself how lucky you are...

Saint Donna

When I was a kid and I'd complain about the soup being too hot after burning the roof of my mouth, my mom, whose name was Donna, would always respond, "Well, you wouldn't want cold soup, would you?" Obviously, gazpacho wasn't big in our house.

My mother was a saint. I know everyone says that about their moms, but my mom really was as good as she seemed. She was unfailingly optimistic and accepting of life as it was. Nothing was *ever* as bad as it seemed; she could find the silver lining in any rain cloud. A Midwest farm girl who grew up during the Depression, she knew what it was like to do without. Her family used to make their own soap with leftover fat drippings! But you never met a happier, more positive, and more kindhearted lady.

When she was in her early sixties, ready to set sail into retirement with my dad—a retirement they had earned through a life of hard work and sacrifice—she was diagnosed with MS. As a result, Mediterranean cruises were exchanged for conversion vans with ramps and motorized wheelchairs. The pain and suffering this woman endured over the next twenty years was hard for me to watch. I knew her as the willowy, active woman she'd always been when I was growing up. Yet she never once complained. Ever. When she lost the ability to walk, she'd show off her motorized chair: "Look what this baby can do." When she lost the use of her right arm: "Oh well, I've still got my left arm." And on and on it went. She was like the Black Knight from *Monty Python and the Holy Grail*. Everything was just a flesh wound. Nothing was ever as bad as it seemed. I have derived so much inspiration from her life. Even in her darkest hour, she saw only light. And that light, I am convinced, propelled her to an eternal life free of wheel-chairs and suffering.

9

SHORT GAME IS EVERYTHING

If you want to understand human nature, just visit your local driving range. You'll see row after row of people wailing away with their drivers. It's an all-you-can-eat "big dog" buffet. And yet, as every golfer knows, it's your short game that has the greatest impact on your score. Sure, thumping it 280 yards down the middle gives you an advantage. And we all know "Chicks dig the long ball." But sixty percent of your strokes are made with a putter. On the PGA Tour, if you don't convert fifty percent of your putts from inside ten feet, you go hungry. It's obvious that the surest, fastest way to lower your handicap is to focus on your short game. Yet most of us continue to grip it and rip it. Chipping and putting just isn't as sexy and fun as trying to blast balls over the net at the end of the driving range.

The same can be true in life. It's easy to become consumed with the power game. The fancy title. The big house. Adding another zero to your net worth. Yet who we are and how we are judged comes down to all the little things we do. Especially when nobody's looking.

Mother Teresa famously said, "I don't do great things. I do small things with great love." I'm guessing Saint Teresa of Calcutta probably never teed it up on a golf course, but if she had, I'm confident she would have been tremendous with the flat stick. Her entire life was devoted to performing small, simple acts of love and compassion. And yet, look what it added up to—sainthood! Just slightly more impressive than a 350-yard drive.

I've enjoyed modest success in life by society's standards. But cancer has given me a new perspective on how I can achieve greater fulfillment. And it's not by attempting to do great things. Now more than ever, I'm focused on my short game: little everyday gestures that I'm convinced make a big difference in the grand scheme of life.

The following are a few examples:

Letting cars merge in front of me in traffic

Really, other than running late for a tee time, where are you going that's so important you can't afford to be polite and allow someone the privilege of sliding into traffic in front of you? I try to provide a nice wide berth so there's no question as to my intentions. I'll even smile and gesture the way a restaurant maître d' might when showing you to your table. This simple act teaches me the importance of generosity. It also stops me from being in such a hurry all the time—a condition that heaps unnecessary stress on our already stressful lives.

Hitting the open button on elevators to allow that straggler on

When I do this, the straggler is always incredibly thankful, and that makes me feel awesome. I'm also making a human connection, which seems to be in decline these days. Next time you're on a crowded elevator, look around and you'll see what I mean. Everybody's on their phones, avoiding eye contact with people at all costs.

Picking up litter in public and properly disposing of it

If you saw garbage on the floor of your house, you'd pick it up, right? Why not in public? The reactions I get from people are funny. They look as shocked as if I had been the person discarding the trash in the first place. Obviously, they've never seen that famous TV commercial from the seventies with the crying Native American.

Smiling at everyone I encounter

This makes me feel like a positive force of nature. Smiling feels great. And the recipients of my free smiles almost always smile back, which feels even better. I especially go out of my way to smile at those on the lower rungs of the socioeconomic ladder.

Walking patiently behind elderly people

Similar to the traffic example, this practice forces you to slow down and breathe easier, which alleviates stress—something I consider as detrimental to health as smoking. And besides, with any luck, this'll be you someday. Wouldn't you appreciate a little patience and understanding from those around you?

Random acts of kindness

Not long ago, I was using the ATM in my office building when I noticed someone had walked away without their cash, a hundred dollars to be exact. I removed it from the machine and quickly went in search of its owner. Not finding anyone, I went back to the ATM and camped out, figuring the owner would eventually realize their mistake and come back. I waited for about five minutes, and just as I was about to give up (I was now in danger of being late for an appointment), I noticed a man with the distinctive look of someone who just left a hundred bucks in a cash machine. I approached him and produced the hundred dollars to his surprise and relief.

It would have been so easy for me to quickly conclude the owner of the cash was long gone and move on with my busy life—a hundred bucks richer! But I didn't. Now I know this hardly puts me in the company of Mother Teresa, but it sure made me feel good. And I can't help but think that forgetful man might one day remember the episode and go out of his way to help someone else.

Like any behavior, the more you perform these little acts, the more they become habit. If everyone was focused on their short game—doing little things with great love—imagine what a better place the world would be? Better yet, let's stop imagining.

PART TWO

THE BACK NINE

10

NO RISK, NO REWARD

In August 2017, my good friend Mark graciously invited me to play in his golf club's invitational tournament, even though I was not in the best shape physically. For the previous nine months, I had been participating in a clinical trial at the University of Minnesota where I underwent drug infusions every other week. I should point out the club he belongs to, Spring Hill, is fairly well known for having a membership made up of captains of industry, sports celebrities, and other assorted alpha males. I only bring this up to point out their invitational is more than a little competitive.

I declined to play in the practice round because I didn't think there'd be enough gas left in the tank to finish the tournament if I did. This turned out to be the right decision. We began play on Friday morning.

I was nearly late for our opening nine-hole four-ball match and flubbed my way through the first few holes, essentially forcing Mark to play solo. Gradually, I settled down, got in the groove and my play improved. Fast forward to Saturday afternoon when, lo and behold, we wound up coming from behind in our final match and won our flight by half a point!

Onto the twelve-team shootout. After barely surviving the first hole in a chip-off, we cruised through the second hole when Mark hit a perfect 9-iron on the par-3 17th hole to twenty feet. I putted to gimme range, and we were off to the final hole with just two other teams remaining. The 18th hole at Spring Hill is a pretty demanding par-4 dogleg left with the driving range and OB left and woods right. I said to Mark, "I'll just hit my hybrid to make sure I get something in the fairway." I figured there's no sense in risking a wild swing with a driver at this point in the proceedings. Let the other guys make a mistake, and we'll capitalize. But Mark would have none of it. He pulled the driver out of my bag, looked me in the eyes and said, "I want you to hit this thing as hard as you f*cking can down the right side." Driver it is!

I've never been a particularly reliable driver of the golf ball. Irons are my strong suit. In fact, I used to hit a 3-iron off the tee most of the time at my home club. But inspired by Mark's "pep talk," I stepped up to the challenge and smoked a nice high draw that started down the right side of the fairway and ended up smack dab in the middle of the fairway. Mark hit next—a 9-iron approach, which he easily landed on the front of the green. This left us with a tricky uphill-downhill forty-footer. The hole was in the very back of the green, and the last ten feet are extremely quick. It's not out of the question that you could putt it off the green. After stalking it for several seconds, I hit my putt, which first appeared as if it might come up well short. But after cresting the upslope, it gained momentum and kept creeping closer and closer to the hole. A murmur went up from the gallery, crescendoing to a full roar as the ball barely missed the lip before finally coming to rest a couple feet past the hole. If you had given me ten tries, I don't think I could have gotten it any closer. Mark easily knocked in our short par putt, and after our competitors could manage no better than bogey, we were the Founder's Cup champions.

Life is a series of challenges in which you have to decide: am I going to play it safe, or am I going to pull driver and go for it? There are countless famous quotations on this subject. "No guts, no glory." "A ship is safe in a harbor, but that is not what ships are for." I can't think of a single quotation encouraging people to play it safe.

When I was a kid, I was pretty shy and introverted. Like a lot of people, I was afraid to put myself out there, open myself up to criticism or ridicule. It wasn't until I discovered music that things changed. I was something of a child prodigy trumpet player. My band directors would always feature me during concerts. Standing up in front of an auditorium filled with people filled me with courage. Through high school and college, I started to put myself out there more and more: running for student government, writing opinion pieces in the student newspaper, asking girls who were well above my social strata to dances. The more I took on, the more I realized that taking chances is integral to finding fulfillment in life.

Throughout our lives, we're frequently asked to volunteer for things. And when those things involve doing something outside our comfort zone, we tend to say no or come up with excuses why we shouldn't say yes. We think we're unworthy, lacking the right skills. We're afraid we'll fail. But if we simply allow ourselves to be used as God's instrument, we learn we're more capable than we ever imagined. Over time, we become fearless. We understand we could choose to hit hybrid and not screw it up, but we also know it wouldn't be nearly as gratifying as pulling out the driver and giving it a rip.

11

THE RIGHT CADDIE MAKES ALL
THE DIFFERENCE

In the fall of 2013, a couple years before my cancer diagnosis, I went on the golf trip of a lifetime with a group of friends to Ireland. We played fourteen rounds in nine days on the finest courses around Dublin and Northern Ireland, including Royal County Down, considered the #1 golf course in the world outside of the United States, and Royal Portrush, home of the 2019 Open Championship. It was at Royal Portrush that I had a chance encounter with a caddie named Rory who would become something of a legend among my friends.

At the time of our trip, I was a nine handicap. But with Rory on my bag, I played almost like a scratch golfer. I don't know what it was about him, but we just clicked. My friends called him "The Doug Whisperer." He was unusually tall for an Irishman (a head taller than me and I'm six-two) with giant ears and an incredibly quiet, gentle demeanor. We spoke sparingly to one another. But it was like we shared an unspoken language. He'd pull clubs, and I'd hit them without question. He'd point to a spot on the green, and I'd putt at it. Whenever I had a short putt for par, he'd say to me, almost in a whisper, "All right, Doug. Show me your confidence." And every time, I'd drill the putt. He knew how to bring out the best in me. And I didn't want to disappoint him.

If you've ever played golf in Ireland, you know the caddies often wager with one another on the players they're caddying for. At one point late in the round, after I flushed another drive right down the middle of the fairway en route to my third birdie, one of the other caddies said, above his breath but just loud enough for us to hear, "No *fooking* way he's a nine!" To this day, it's the single highest compliment anyone's ever paid my golf game. In incredibly windy and difficult conditions, I ended up bogeying the final two holes and shooting 80.

My friends still bring up Rory and my unforgettable round at Royal Portrush. We even joked about flying Rory to Minneapolis so he could caddie for me in our club's Member/Member tournament. Rory serves as a constant reminder to me that there's incredible strength that can be derived from human connections and relying on others.

Most people, men especially, have a hard time coming to terms with this. It's at odds with the American "rugged individualism" ethos. We're taught to be independent, take responsibility. Relying on others might be viewed as a sign of weakness.

I'll be the first to admit I have a healthy ego and a high degree of confidence in my abilities. But cancer has reminded me of my frailty, and that ultimately, I need to rely on the grace of others, including my medical team and my incredible friends and family. This doesn't make me feel weak. On the contrary, the more I rely on the healing power of community, the stronger I feel. I know that, come what may, I'll never be alone, and all will be well.

But What About When You Get the Wrong Caddie?

When I was first diagnosed with bladder cancer, I was seeing a urologist who was plenty competent, but I just wasn't feeling the love, so I switched to a new doctor. A generation ago, most people would never consider doing this. Medicine was so shrouded in mystery, people would never second-guess or take issue with the recommendations of someone who had gone to school for eight years. But today, we understand the most important member of your care team is you. Not to mention it's so easy to research doctors and treatment options online. Who you pick for your care team is critically important to your health, not only physically but emotionally as well. You're going to be spending a lot of time with them. It's important they bring good energy.

Hope Rx

In talking to other cancer survivors, I have determined the strongest cancer drug available is hope. For some people, it might be hope in possibility. For me, it's hope in God. There's a Gospel reading in which Luke compares our relationship with God to a tree planted near a river. Because of this relationship, even in drought conditions, our leaves remain green, and our branches continue to bear fruit. What a simple, powerful metaphor. And what a comfort to know that God is always present to us, even when we're not present to God. You might say God is like the ultimate caddie. He lightens your load, shows you the lines, helps you avoid the hazards, inspires you with confidence, and never stops loving and believing in you. With someone like that on your bag, you can overcome a lot.

12

OWN YOUR SWING

A lot of amateur golfers try to emulate the swings of professional tour players. In fact, this has become a popular teaching method, where golf instructors will make a video of your golf swing and show it side by side with the swing of a PGA Tour player with a similar body type to yours.

It all makes perfect sense. A picture is worth a thousand words. And besides, we learn things like speech and language from imitating others. Why not swinging a golf club?

The challenge comes when you're in your fifties and you're trying to imitate the swing of a flat-bellied twenty-something who has the flexibility of a willow branch. It's a great way to end up in the orthopedic surgeon's office.

And while there are lessons to be gleaned from studying the swings of others, the fact is, there's no one else quite like you, for better or worse. So I say, to thine own swing be true!

Just look at professional golfers like Jim Furyk, Bubba Watson, Lee Trevino, even Arnold Palmer. Every one of them had a golf swing as unique as their fingerprint. And yet they all went on to have all-star careers.

There was a great commercial for Dick's Sporting Goods several years ago. It featured golfers of all shapes and sizes swinging in each person's inimitable style. The narrator was none other than Arnold Palmer, and the spot culminated with an old black-and-white clip of the King and his signature chicken wing follow-through.

Arnold Palmer: Swing your swing. Not some idea of a swing. Not a swing you saw on TV. Not that swing you wish you had. No, swing your swing. Capable of greatness. Prized only by you. Perfect in its imperfection. Swing your swing. I know I did.

Exploring the You-niverse

I believe God truly wants us to be happy. That's why he endowed us with certain gifts and characteristics shared by nobody else, that we might leverage those gifts in ways that bring us joy and God greater glory.

The trick is discovering what those gifts are. This comes easier for some than others: the child prodigy musician, the natural athlete, the gifted math student. Others' gifts might be more hidden or take longer to uncover.

Too often, the individual is inclined to bow to society's expectations. The world is full of miserable doctors, lawyers, and bankers who were never meant to be any of those things. The good news is, it's never too late to let your true light shine. A friend of mine who had a very successful career in marketing got out of the business in his fifties and started a tree-trimming service, an occupation that aligned with his deep desire to pursue an occupation more connected to the land. John Grisham, before he went on to publishing fame, was a lawyer who grew up wanting to be a baseball player.

Different Is Good

It truly does take all kinds. And we should be receptive, even appreciative of those who are "unique." Or as we say in Minnesota, where passive-aggressive behavior has been raised to an art form, "different."

My wife, Michaelanne, threw a big party for me when I turned forty. What I remember most about that evening was the eclectic assortment of people in attendance. There were my liberal advertising friends, my conservative country club friends, my guy's-guy college friends, my long-haired musician friends, my polite church friends. When asked to give a speech, I joked about how great it was to see all my blue and red state friends in the same room having a great time. Our world has become so polarized, especially politically. It doesn't have to be that way. If we developed more of an appreciation for diversity, we'd fight less.

I do draw the line somewhere. My brother Dan, who's a huge Jimmy Buffett fan, has this humongous "Margaritaville" golf bag complete with a colorfully embroidered parrot on the side. I keep hoping the airlines will lose it at some point.

Dear Harry...

My son, Harry, was born with a rare condition: his looks and mannerisms are freakishly similar to mine. I mentioned him earlier in this book as having had some fairly serious health issues in his late teens. He's twenty-four now and in very good health. My friends often refer to him as "Mini-Doug." He started off at the University of Missouri School of Journalism wanting to become a sportscaster, but then he switched to advertising—my business for the past thirty years. I tried to talk him out of it, but he was determined. He currently works for a well-known customer loyalty marketing firm and seems to be doing well. I suspect he looks up to me in the way most sons look up to their fathers. That said, I sincerely hope I'm not his measuring stick. I want him to carve out his own niche in the world. Optimize his many unique gifts. Swing his own swing.

13

IT'S ALL IN YOUR HEAD

If you've never had the putting yips, count yourself lucky. There is no swing malady more mysterious or debilitating. Your hands flinch uncontrollably at impact, causing you to miss putts you'd normally make in your sleep. You'll try anything to cure them. The hard part is, unlike a slice or a hook, which are the result of physical flaws, the yips are entirely mental. Or at least, I think they are.

I developed the yips not long after undergoing chemotherapy. Part of me wonders if the two events weren't related; chemo can be pretty hard on nerve endings. Two-footers, which I used to bang against the back of the cup, now made my knees shake. As painful as it was to experience, it was equally painful to watch. I had to warn people to look away when I was putting.

I tried everything to fix it. Going to a shorter, quicker stroke; a slower, longer stroke; eyes on the hole; eyes closed; left hand low; claw grip; pencil grip; long putter; short putter; fat grip; skinny grip. These tricks provided nothing more than short-term relief, then the yips would return. The best I could hope for was I'd get the ball close enough to the hole that someone would give me the putt. This continued on and off for several years. Then one day, I stopped thinking about them, and the yips more or less went away.

The control our minds have over our bodies is real, yet not very well understood. Which is why, when my wife signed me up for a session with a Reiki healer shortly after my cancer diagnosis, I said, "Great!" I didn't even ask, "What's a Reiki healer?" I just showed up at this complete stranger's house, where he took me to this tiny room in his basement that looked like an Eastern religious shrine. In the middle of the room was a massage table tented off with white muslin fabric. He explained the basic concept of Reiki, which was developed in Japan in the early twentieth century. It involves a technique called "hands-on healing," through which a universal energy is said to be transferred through the palms of the practitioner to the patient in order to encourage emotional or physical healing. He'd place his hands over my seven chakras, not touching my body but hovering just above it, and this would somehow remove negative energy. He also offered to "channel me," which I politely declined.

Needless to say, this is pretty exotic stuff for a registered Republican. But I wasn't willing to leave any money on the table. Cancer is a zero-sum game. Even if you get rid of 99% of the cancer, you'll still end up 100% dead. As with the yips, I was willing to try anything. Besides, I don't believe that surgery and drugs are the answer to every medical problem. Even if there is no empirical evidence of the healing powers of Reiki, I did find the whole experience incredibly peaceful and relaxing. And what could be wrong with that? At the end of my session, even though I requested not to be channeled, he did share one observation: He said I needed to pay closer attention to signs in my life. Ooo-kay.

A few months later, I was meeting up with my friend Tom at our golf club. It was right after I got my chemo cut, or as my barber calls it, "Taking it down to the wood." We were sitting in the bar, and people were approaching me, curious to know why I suddenly looked like Stewart Cink. Before I could explain, you could tell by the suddenly somber expressions on their faces that they had figured it out. I matter-of-factly explained my situation, told them it was no big deal, that I had a plan in place, and everything was under control. Their moods instantly bounced back.

Tom, who had a front-row seat as I soldiered on through most of my treatments, including this more recent chemo phase, said to me, "Doug, I watch the way you deal with people in light of your illness, and I gotta say, you have a true gift for maintaining a creative posture and staying positive. And I see the way it rubs off on people. I believe a lot of people could benefit from hearing you tell your story."

Maybe this was one of the signs the Reiki healer was telling me about. Regardless, it is one of the reasons I decided to write this book.

14

TECHNOLOGY, THE GREAT GAME CHANGER

It doesn't seem like it was that many years ago we were all swatting rubber band-filled balata golf balls with persimmon wood drivers. In fact, TaylorMade's metal driver didn't really become mainstream until the late eighties. Davis Love III, one of the last holdouts on Tour, was still using a persimmon driver as recently as 1997!

The difference technology has made in adding distance and improving accuracy is nothing short of revolutionary. In 1980, which is the first year the PGA Tour's driving distance stats are available, the Tour average was a whopping 257 yards per drive. Today, it's 295 yards. And distances continue to increase every year. Half of this newfound length is coming from club technology. The other half is coming from ball innovations.

Where it stops, nobody knows. Golf courses are now faced with the challenge of keeping up with longer hitters. It used to be that 7,000 yards was considered a long golf course. The 2018 U.S. Open at Shinnecock Hills played to 7,445 yards, par 70!

The same march forward is happening in the treatment of cancer. Over the past few years, chemotherapy and radiation, long considered the gold standard of care, have started to give way to immunotherapy and a new wave of drugs commonly known as checkpoint inhibitors. The way they work and the promise they're showing is remarkable.

An important part of the immune system is its ability to distinguish between normal and foreign cells in the body. This lets the immune system attack foreign cells while leaving normal cells alone. To do this, it uses "checkpoints"—molecules on certain immune cells that need to be activated or inactivated to start an immune response.

Cancer cells sometimes find ways to use these checkpoints to avoid being attacked by the immune system. I liken it to the defense shield in *Star Wars: The Empire Strikes Back*. Immune checkpoint inhibitors lower the shield, so your immune system can go after the evildoers.

I'm living proof of the promise of immunotherapy. I had chemotherapy—the standard of care—before having my bladder and prostate removed. Unfortunately, my cancer didn't respond to it. So, after my disease progressed to stage IV, I was prescribed immunotherapy, which was only covered by insurance because chemotherapy had already been tried and was unsuccessful.

Had I been in this same situation just a year and a half later, my choices would have been totally different. Today, the standard of care recognized by insurance providers includes immunotherapy as a first-line treatment along with chemotherapy. That's a seismic shift, especially when you consider how reluctant insurance companies are to pay for things that are even remotely "experimental."

Whether chemo will go the way of persimmon is too early to tell. As promising as immunotherapy is, the success metrics are far from a slam dunk. As I mentioned earlier in this book, Keytruda, the drug I was on, has a response rate of just twenty-nine percent.

15

GO WITH THE FLOW

Ever have one of those career rounds going where you're cruising along at or under par with just a few holes to play, and then you make the fatal mistake—you remind yourself that you're at or under par with just a few holes to play?! You know what happens next. You start thinking. Your swing, which had been syrupy-smooth, begins to tighten up and become mechanical, even defensive. Your pulse rate quickens. Your posture sags. In the words of Austin Powers, "You've lost your mojo!"

Johnny Miller, one of the greats on the links and in the broadcast booth, was very candid about calling out tour players when they choked. He readily admitted that he himself had been guilty of choking on more than one occasion, which lent credence to his blunt analysis.

It goes to show how fragile the mind can be. When you're "feeling it," you're simply going with the flow. It's a Zen-like experience. But when you engage your brain, all hell breaks loose. It takes you out of your rhythm.

Holistic healers talk about mindfulness, which is a misnomer, because the purpose of mindfulness is to not have anything on your mind, to just be present in the moment. This again is one of the goals of meditation— to rid the mind of conscious thought and the stress it can create.

For the record, I have found Hamm's beer to help restore flow. Although my oncologist would not like me sharing this advice.

Slow. Down.

Breathing is an important aspect of golf that pros work really hard on. It's important because it helps them stay calm in stressful situations. You never see them rush between shots. They're always relaxed, measured, methodical, going with the flow.

We could all benefit from applying this to everyday life. Our world continues to spin faster and faster, which makes us more and more impatient. Few of us come to a complete stop at stop signs anymore. When an internet app doesn't open the second we click on it, we're outraged—never mind the fact that the technology only recently came into being, and it's light years faster than the previous technology!

Life isn't a race. And even if it was, do you really want to reach the finish line first?

All this impatience causes stress, which many experts believe is a major contributor to inflammation and illness. You're no doubt familiar with the fight-or-flight response. When we're in danger, a stress hormone called cortisol is released in our bodies that enables us to escape. The more frequently the fight-or-flight response is activated, the more likely it is to be activated again. What's more, it'll take less to activate it, and the response will be more forceful. It's like when you're running late for an appointment and already stressed, then someone slows down in front of you, and you completely freak out.

Our cars are death traps. Not so much because of the physical injury risk they pose, but because of the stress they create. Otherwise kind, gentle souls get into their cars and turn into crazed lunatics. I used to be that guy who'd race to the four-way stop so I could go first. But cancer has convinced me to slow down. Now I'm one of those weirdos who gently comes to a complete stop. And I mean complete. I could be holding a cup of hot coffee without a lid and I wouldn't spill. There's a sensation you get from coming to a complete stop that's almost therapeutic. It's like hitting the pause button on life. The world stops spinning for a brief moment and breathes a sigh of relief. Seriously! Try it sometime and you'll know exactly what I mean. The best part is, it snowballs, influencing your behavior the rest of the day. You become less hurried, which helps restore flow.

16

YOU'RE NEVER OUT OF IT

You've no doubt heard people describe "Ray-Ray" rounds—ones in which they played like Ray Charles on the front nine and Ray Floyd on the back. I'm sure we can all point to similar rounds that started inauspiciously enough, only to finish brilliantly. As I mentioned in the introduction, the best round of golf I ever played started with a double bogey.

When I first received the news of my cancer diagnosis, I thought, why couldn't I expect the same amazing turnaround? Why couldn't my diagnosis, while as unwelcome as the shanks, lead to something great?

Of course, you say that to yourself. But it's another thing to make it happen. We've all started a round poorly before. And by the fourth or fifth hole, we're veritably sprinting to the clubhouse to get it over with.

Throwing in the towel isn't an option with cancer, at least one that doesn't involve an early grave. So you've got to find a way to erase the first hole from your memory bank and get busy finding the bottom of the cup.

Some people are better at moving past adversity than others. We all know our share of pessimists and malcontents. Theirs is an inability to shake the Etch A Sketch and move on.

It's not easy to forget you have cancer, especially if you're in the treatment phase and spending a lot of time in cancer clinic waiting rooms surrounded by other people with cancer. However, I've found ways to trick my mind. One is by making plans for the future. Some of the plans I make are ambitious, as if I'm planning on living forever. This is the opposite of Jesse Helms, the 90-something North Carolina senator, who would joke, "At my age, I don't even order room service."

Full disclosure: I wasn't always capable of thinking this way. Early on, my thought process was more pragmatic: I thought I probably wasn't long for this world, so maybe I should start thinking about early retirement and checking items off my bucket list.

I'm still thinking about early retirement from the ad agency world. But not so I can crank out wooden birdhouses in my wood shop, which I don't even have. My plan is to build other things, to take the skills I've gained from a lifetime in advertising and apply them to causes that might in some small way make the world a better place. "He was a creative force for good." That's what I want written on my tombstone. And yes, I would like to devote more time to lowering my handicap.

Music Therapy

My LinkedIn bio reads, "A onetime musical prodigy with perfect pitch, driving quantifiable business results and social change as an award-winning advertising copywriter and creative leader for 30 years." As I mentioned earlier in this book, I was considered a gifted trumpet player in my youth. I still play, but very infrequently, and mostly in the seclusion of my basement.

Last summer, I decided to organize a jazz concert fundraiser for the University of Minnesota Masonic Cancer Center called *Cancer Blows* starring yours truly on trumpet. Joining me on stage was a group of mostly young up-and-coming musicians. It was a true labor of love. I'll toot my own horn and say it took a fair amount of guts and perhaps a large dose of insanity to attempt this. As I said, I don't play much anymore, and trumpet is a physically demanding instrument that requires daily practice to keep up your embouchure, or lip muscles. Needless to say, I was risking making a fool of myself. It did help to be surrounded on stage by musical geniuses. By every measure, the event was a huge success. So much so that we decided to make it an annual event. Any money I might raise pales in comparison to what I've gotten out of it. It's given me another reason to live, which I partially attribute to my still being alive.

In addition to music, I started teaching an advertising class at my alma mater, the University of St. Thomas in St. Paul, Minnesota. I'm involved in helping an up-and-coming clothing retail brand with their marketing. I've even toyed around with the idea of becoming a farmer. Although, the chances of getting Michaelanne to go along with me on this venture are about as good as my chances of making it on the PGA Champions Tour. I'm picturing scenes from "Green Acres."

Are there times when I'm reminded of the fact that my cancer might suddenly return? I'd be lying if I said there weren't. But the more I occupy my mind with proactive, creative thoughts, the easier it is to forget about it. In fact, I recently needed to decide whether to have my IV port surgically removed, or leave it in, in the event I need more treatments. Duh. That baby's coming out.

17

NUTRITION—THE FIFTEENTH CLUB IN THE BAG

I love watching old footage of golf tournaments on the Golf Channel, from the classic reverse-C golf swings of guys like Johnny Miller to the swashbuckling antics of characters like Lee Trevino and Seve Ballesteros. And then there are the body types. No wonder Sansabelt slacks were so popular back then; the bellies were as prodigious as the bell-bottoms. And how about the number of golfers who smoked. On television!

It's not that golf wasn't considered a sport back in the days of Craig "The Walrus" Stadler, but players spent a lot more time in the buffet line than they did on the elliptical. And the idea of working with a strength coach? Yeah, right.

Even after factoring for technology advancements, golfers today hit the ball a mile farther than golfers of the past, for obvious reasons. Today's average golfer is leaner, stronger, more flexible. This is all largely the result of a great awakening in health, fitness, and nutrition. We're much more knowledgeable about the role of food in our overall health, as well as the importance of maintaining muscle strength and elasticity to avoid injury.

Of course, it takes a ton of discipline to avoid weighing a ton. After all, we live in a "more culture." Look at some of the fast food ads on TV. The hamburgers look like they were constructed with a crane: three beef patties piled high with bacon, onion straws, an egg, and half a quart of barbecue sauce. It's not so much food as it is a dare.

The statistics around obesity in the U.S. are alarming. According to the Centers for Disease Control and Prevention, nearly forty percent of adults had obesity in 2016, compared to roughly thirty percent in 2000. In fact, health experts predict obesity will soon surpass smoking as the number one cause of cancer. Of course, you don't need to read these numbers to know something's going on. Just look around. My hometown of Minneapolis is considered one of the healthiest cities in America. And yet every day at lunchtime, I witness scores of people attempting suicide over their lunch break. In one hand is a bag of triple-decker cheeseburgers and curly fries, in the other, a 64-ounce glass of lightly carbonated high fructose corn syrup.

I'm not telling you anything you don't already know. And yet the problem persists. Of course, there have been positive signs in recent years. Kale is trending. Rice bowls and wraps are replacing grease-stained bags from burger joints.

I recognize that food can be an indulgence. I love a good porterhouse as much as the next person. But at its most basic, food is fuel. Put in the proper mix, don't overfill your tank, and your engine will hum.

I confess, I never paid much attention to nutrition before cancer, mostly because I'm one of those terminally skinny people who can eat whatever he wants without gaining weight. That doesn't mean I don't pay attention to what I put in my fuel tank. I'm very good at listening to my body when it tells me I need broccoli or salad. Not to mention that my wife, who's a yoga instructor and a vegetarian, takes very good care of our family, nutritionally and otherwise.

After cancer, I was motivated to learn more about food and its impact on health. I watched documentaries from medical/nutrition experts like Joel Fuhrman and learned new mantras like "The whiter the bread, the quicker you're dead." I started opting for brown instead of white rice and foods made with whole grains. I never had a problem with sugar since I never had much of a sweet tooth. But giving up "distilled sugars" was another story. I've been known to partake of a little scotch. Okay, more than a little. I usually had a cocktail every night before dinner. It was part of my evening ritual, and I enjoyed it. But as any nutritionist will tell you, sugar feeds cancer. If you've ever had a PET scan, you know this. PET, which stands for positron-emission tomography, is an imaging technique that is used to observe metabolic processes in the body to help diagnose disease. Before you're scanned, they give you a sugary drink laced with a radioactive isotope. Cancer cells consume eighteen to nineteen times more glucose than healthy cells. All that metabolic activity glows red on a scan, which suggests cancer is present. The cancer cells are like piranhas feeding on the sugar.

I didn't give up alcohol completely, but I reduced my consumption by about seventy-five percent. And when I did, I couldn't believe how quickly the weight started falling off me. Since I didn't need to lose weight, I had to increase my protein intake to compensate. And the best part is, I don't miss alcohol one bit. Not to mention I'm saving a fortune. Alcohol easily accounts for twenty to thirty percent of your restaurant bill. More money for golf.

18

YOU'RE NOT CALLING THE SHOTS

For many years, "You're the man!" was the popular refrain among overzealous fans on the PGA Tour. More recently, it's been replaced by such prosaic genius as "Mashed potato!" and "Baba-booey!" Fueled by testosterone and perhaps a few too many Coors Lights, these primal screams are the ultimate expression of unbridled male aggression. They also suggest that perhaps we're not as far removed from our hairy ancestors as we think.

Our culture is obsessed with winners and "winning." But the fact is, there are so many factors in life we have little control over. Nobody is "the man" after all.

War and Peace

Not long ago, on the Bladder Cancer Advocacy Network website, someone posed the question, "What kind of language do you use to describe your cancer experience?" As you might expect, most people gravitate toward military jargon. They refer to themselves as warriors engaged in a battle in which they're trying to defeat an enemy. And in the end, there will be winners, and there will be losers. Nobody describes going after Alzheimer's this way. But cancer is different; it brings out the alpha in everyone.

While I appreciate the sentiment, I've never embraced the notion of being at war with cancer. I have no desire to carpet bomb my enemy with chemicals and extreme prejudice. In fact, I'm taking the opposite approach: I'm trying to hug it out, not slug it out. How? By eliminating stress, striving for inner peace, practicing better nutrition, redoubling my efforts to put God at the center of my life, and figuring out what he wants me to learn from this experience.

If I live, it's not because I'm a winner. Nor does it mean that I'm a loser if I ultimately succumb to cancer. I'm not suggesting I'm powerless over my health, or that effort and attitude don't play a role in recovery—they most certainly do. I'm also not recommending people forgo traditional western medicine. My point is this: if that's all you're doing, you're only treating the symptom, not the underlying cause. I firmly believe our bodies have the ability to heal themselves, and I'm trying to give mine every opportunity to do just that.

Unlocking the Pharmacy in Your Brain

Every night as I'm lying in bed, I repeat a simple phrase that's become my mantra: "Thank you, God, for the gift of long life." I repeat this several times as I'm dozing off. I'll visualize cancer cells retreating from my body like outgoing waves on the beach. If you've read much on the subject of cancer, you've no doubt learned of others who employ similar visualization techniques.

The mind is a powerful machine. We know so little of its capabilities. Might it be capable of ridding our bodies of disease? I believe it is. How else can you explain the placebo effect? There have been drug studies where patients who received the placebo had better than a fifty percent response rate. Sometimes, they had nearly the same response rate as the people who got the drug. Regardless, if you have a terminal, life-threatening illness, are you so convinced that drugs and radiation are the only solution that you're not willing to at least try less toxic, more holistic alternatives?

Perhaps you've heard of the book Radical Remission and its author, Dr. Kelly Turner. As part of her Ph.D. work, Turner interviewed over a hundred people with metastatic cancer who experienced what's commonly referred to as "spontaneous remission," meaning their cancer just went away with no medical explanation. She wanted to find out what these people had in common that might explain their odds-defying healing. The following are nine factors they shared:

- Radically changed their diet
- Took control of their health
- Followed their intuition
- Used herbs and supplements
- Released suppressed emotions
- Increased positive emotions
- Embraced social support
- Deepened their spiritual connection
- Had a strong reason for living

What's interesting to note is that only two of these characteristics are physical; the rest involve the mind and soul.

Hug It Out, Not Slug It Out

I understand the concept of fighting fire with fire, and that war can sometimes lead to peace. But I also appreciate the wisdom of Dr. Martin Luther King, Jr.:

"Peace cannot be kept by force; it can only be achieved by understanding. Darkness cannot drive out darkness; only light can do that. Hate cannot drive out hate; only love can do that."

I'm reminded of one of my favorite *Aesop's Fables* from childhood, "The North Wind and the Sun." The North Wind challenges the Sun to a competition to find out which one can make a passing traveler remove his cloak. The North Wind blows and blows, but the man only holds on tighter to his cloak to stay warm. But under the Sun's gentle rays, the man becomes warm, removes his cloak, and basks in the glow of the Sun's radiant light.

Hope. Faith. Optimism. Altruism. Charity. Generosity. Love. Humility. The right side of the fairway is lined with these life-affirming values. We know what's on the other side: Despair. Cynicism. Greed. Hatred. Envy. Pride. Narcissism.

My advice: keep it right.

THE 19TH HOLE

I'd like to raise a glass (mine is full of Macallan 18-year, by the way) to all those who've journeyed with me over the past several years, on and off the golf course. I couldn't begin to list you all by name without fear of accidentally omitting someone, so this list of "families" will have to do:

- My Minikahda family
- My Curly Rough family
- My University of St. Thomas family
- My Jefferson High School family
- My Fallon McElligott family
- My Carmichael Lynch family
- My GdB family
- My St. Thomas the Apostle family

- My University of Minnesota Health family, specifically, my medical team:

  - Dr. Badrinath Konety

  - Dr. Chris Weight

  - Dr. Shilpa Gupta

  - Dr. Gautam Jha

  - Dr. Anne-Marie Leuck

  - Kate Boulanger, RN

  - Lucy Reinhardt, PA-C

And, of course, my family family—my wife, Michaelanne; our three children, Harry, Charlie and Gigi; my dad, James deGrood; my seven brothers, Thomas, Richard (Dick), Mark, Dan, Paul, Brian and John; and my one battle-tested sister, Ann

Special thanks to my editors, Patricia Weaver Francisco and Sarah Howard.

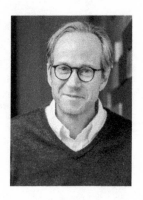

ABOUT THE AUTHOR

In addition to an avid golfer and stage IV bladder cancer survivor, Doug deGrood has been a fixture in the Minneapolis advertising community for going on three decades. A copywriter and creative director, he was one of the founding partners of boutique agency Gabriel deGrood Bendt. This is his first published work, unless you count the hundreds of ads he's created.

DeGrood lives in Edina, Minnesota, with his wife, Michaelanne. Together, they have three adult children; Harry, Charlie, and Gigi; an old black cat named Alice; and a pug dog named Birdie. He is a member of the Minikahda Club in Minneapolis, where he recently served as the club's grounds chairperson.

At the time this book went to press, Mr. deGrood learned his cancer had relapsed. He has vowed to birdie the next hole.